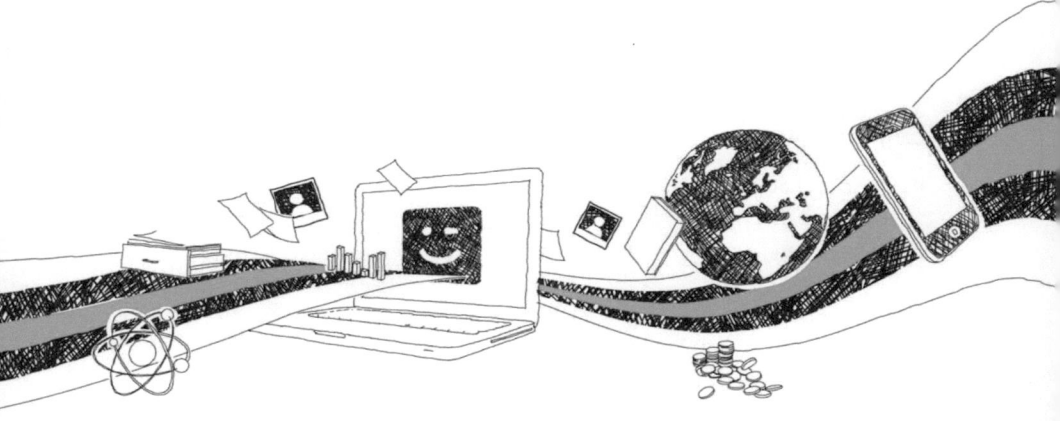
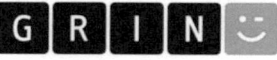

**Bibliographic information published by the German National Library:**

The German National Library lists this publication in the National Bibliography; detailed bibliographic data are available on the Internet at http://dnb.dnb.de .

**Imprint:**

Copyright © 2015 GRIN Verlag, Open Publishing GmbH
Print and binding: Books on Demand GmbH, Norderstedt Germany
ISBN: 978-3-668-02899-9

**This book at GRIN:**

http://www.grin.com/en/e-book/303357/kuwait-paramedic-preparedness-to-mass-casualty-and-terrorism

Ahmad Al Harbi

# Kuwait Paramedic Preparedness to Mass Casualty and Terrorism

GRIN Publishing

**GRIN - Your knowledge has value**

Since its foundation in 1998, GRIN has specialized in publishing academic texts by students, college teachers and other academics as e-book and printed book. The website www.grin.com is an ideal platform for presenting term papers, final papers, scientific essays, dissertations and specialist books.

**Visit us on the internet:**

http://www.grin.com/

http://www.facebook.com/grincom

http://www.twitter.com/grin_com

# Kuwait Paramedic Preparedness to Mass Casualty and

# Terrorism

Ahmad ALHarbi

Phd .Emergency Services Management
Master Degree in Health Professions Education
Bachelor Degree in Clinical Practice(Paramedics)

**Kuwait Paramedic Preparedness to Mass Casualty and Terrorism**

The level of uncertainty that characterizes the world today makes it almost impossible to tell what might happen the next minute. The threat of terrorism is as real as ever, and no one knows when and where terrorists will strike next. Global warming has increased to such a level that natural disasters like floods or tsunamis are what make news every day. More than ever before, a need arises to have in place efficient medical emergency services that should have the capacity to handle mass casualties that may result out of the mentioned disasters or terrorist attacks. Oftentimes, putting in place such healthcare and emergency response systems has been the duty of governments, although local, regional, and international organizations have also continued to play a vital role. Sometimes it has emerged to be more fruitful when there are combined efforts between such organizations and the governments of countries where they operate. International co-operation and support has also proved to be imperative. This construction discusses the preparedness of the Kuwait's emergency medical services as far as paramedic response to risks of mass casualty and terrorism are concerned.

First, it is imperative to note that Kuwait's geographical position makes it prone to risks of terrorism. This gulf country shares borders with Iran and Iraq, both high profile countries as regards possible terror attacks (Alexander, 2007). This calls for adequate preparedness to handle developments that may result in loss of lives or major/minor injuries to many people. Otherwise, a direct implication would be the unimaginable overwhelming of the country's medical emergency health service in particular and the healthcare system in general in the event of a large-scale terror attack. In the same manner, natural disasters could strike and the thought of what could happen without adequate preparedness is appalling. It is therefore very important to ensure that the emergency medical services are not strained and that there are minimal casualties.

The threat of terror becomes more vivid with the comprehension of the role that Kuwait has assumed in the war against terrorism. Since January 2005, the country's government forces have engaged in close to ten terror firefights with terrorist cells (Boghard, 2006). The country's role in the global war on terror was a hitherto low-profile issue but since military operations begun in Iraq, it has been brought to the fore. Related developments have magnified the terrorist threat that the country faces.  More precisely, Kuwait hosts servicemen in the figure of 37,500 besides military contractors involved in various operations in Iraq. It has also become a major center of attraction for usual commercial contingent expatriates from Western countries. These are all major targets for jihadists operating in the region. To understand how the terror threat has developed in Kuwait, one notes that quite a small minority of the country's citizens have continuously demonstrated their intent to engage in acts of Islamic militancy (Alexander, 2007). However, such elements have lacked the capability to the effect of undertaking serious activities of terror, as they have remained largely cut from the larger jihadist network. This is because radicals and mosques alike have been put under tight surveillance. Consequently, young Kuwaitis motivated by news coverage of the Israeli-Palestinian and Iraq conflicts to engage in violent activities of terror have not been able to make contact with the wider Al Qaeda network, let alone with each other. Terror cells in Kuwait have been able to achieve what is referred to as 'articulation' in terrorism analysis circles (Cordesman, & Gold, 2014). This term is employed in reference to the development of special units or cells each tasked with financing, bombarding or planning the attacks. In other instances, isolated and scattered groups have formed their own units and as such strike haphazardly using whichever weapons they may have at hand. Such has oftentimes led to a rash of shootings with many casualties. An incident of such nature culminated in the court martial of some Kuwaiti officers taken into custody in December 2004 and charged with plotting to kill American soldiers during a joint maneuver of U.S. and Kuwaiti troops (Terril, & Army War College, 2007). A lesson drawn from here is that there is need for adequate medical emergency preparedness since anyone can be targeted.

Authorities in Kuwait seem to be much aware of this terrorism threat and a possible occurrence of other natural incidents that are likely to lead to mass casualties. For this reason, the country boasts of one of the best ambulance services in the Gulf region. The Emergency Medical Service (EMS) attracts attention in this regard and qualifies for an in-depth exploration as regards preparedness to deal with natural disasters or incidents of terror that are likely to affect scores of people once they occur. The ambulance service's central Control Center is situated in Subhan.

The need for an efficient medical emergency service in Kuwait necessitated the demolition and rebuilding of the EMS's Control Center anew, thus yielding the most developed state of the art system in the entire Gulf region (Abbas, 1999). It is responsible and obligated to dispatch ambulances in events of emergency. One wonders; how effective is the system? What happens when news of unfolding disastrous events are received? Indeed, there is a lot that happens behind the scenes at the control center that could gain relevance in the discussion of how prepared the country is to handle emergencies as in the context under discussion. When one places a call to the emergency hotline (112), they would be in essence forwarding their call to the Control Center of EMS. Now, the ambulance service's objective is to have an ambulance reach the location of interest under 8 minutes. This is not just a dream goal on paper but something they must achieve no matter the location within Kuwait. Whether one is in Failaka and requests for an emergency they shall get the same within 8 minutes. Even in worst-case scenarios where there has been an explosion for instance, and perhaps people buried under rubble and many need urgent medical attention, EMS gets an ambulance to the scene under the said time. The system is as efficient as has been witnessed in the past. Its workability is a central point of interest that would help gain insight and understanding on how the wider medical emergency service system in Kuwait is prepared to handle mass casualty and terrorism-related incidents that could result to the same.

The EMS Control Center comprises of three groups all sitting in the department. They do so in three rows. They can be listed as the Call Takers, the Dispatchers, and the Supervisors. When one calls EMS or gets their call forwarded to the center, the call is received by a Call Taker who then communicates with the Dispatcher to whom he passes the information regarding the situation on the ground as may be received from the caller. After receiving the call and establishing contact with the Dispatcher, he stays on the line to keep getting updated information from the ground as well as pass on instructions on what needs to be done to keep the situation in check before help arrives (Abbas, 1999). In front of them are screens showing information such as the phone number and call history. Onto one of the screens is where the Call Taker fills in information like the kind of event that occurred, location or physical address of the event as well as caller information. In addition, one of the screens has a map of Kuwait that keeps updating live zooming depending on the location that has been inputted in the other screen. Take for instance a situation where there is a fire outbreak in a densely populated town in central Kuwait, and then an explosion is reported near the border with Iraq; the screen specified for live updates will update the information but still keep signaling on all affected areas. This acts as a reminder in case previous events have not been exhaustively dealt with.

It is imperative to note that the system is automated and highly efficient. For this reason it has proved useful in more ways than one in avoiding mass casualties and initiating response whenever terrorist activities have occurred. One of its most unique qualities that make it efficient is the fact that it pinpoints location and leads dispatched rescuers to the location of the event or incident. What if the caller reporting an incident does not know the exact location of the place where help is needed? In such a case, the EMS uses known landmarks. For instance if there has been a fire or terrorist attack at Sultan Center and the caller dials from Salmiya, the EMS operator can type Sultan Center  and additionally the area near Salmiya after which it shall be displayed on the map. When an event of interest takes place in an area that has no landmarks nearby, callers are instructed to locate nearest lampposts and read the indicated numbers to the EMS operators. Assuming one is on the highway en route to Wafra and a tanker transporting oil catches fire it may be very difficult for one to state their exact location since much of the surrounding area is empty desert. This is where lampposts gain relevance since the numbers on them can be used by the EMS to locate the exact location of the incident or accident. After establishing the exact location of interest, the Call Taker sends the same to the Dispatchers, a step that prompts a new screen to pop up. This contains instructions that the Call Taker reads to the caller and guides them on what should or should not be done as help is being awaited. The Call Taker can end the call after a rescue team and ambulance arrives. One notes here that most of the time the people who call are in a state of shock or panic and only a slight percentage actually listens or follows instructions.

On the other hand, Dispatchers set things rolling behind the scenes after being alerted by the Call Takers. While the Call Takers maintain contact with the callers and get updates from the ground even as they issue instructions, the Dispatchers work in the background and make every effort to see that ambulances get to the location of the caller within the shortest time possible, usually targeted at less than 8 minutes. Their set up is similar to that of the Call Takers, only that theirs has additional features. For instance, they are able to visually see locations of all ambulances within Kuwait along with additional information on every available ambulance like their current location and travel speed. Once a Call Taker informs a Dispatcher about an unfolding event, a freaky and annoying Siren goes off in the entire department thus alerting all Dispatchers about the event, incident, or accident. The siren only goes off after the Dispatcher has accepted the event on their screen.

What does the Dispatcher do after being notified of an event? First, he alerts all the ambulances in the area concerning the incident. He then sends the same information to the Regional Ambulance Center. It is noted here that Kuwait has been divided into six parts and each part has its own Ambulance Center. The system has been digitalized and fitted with the latest technology with each Ambulance served with a laptop, and once they receive notification of the event, the one that replies first takes the rescue/help mission. If it so happens that within two minutes no ambulance answers the event, the Dispatcher is alerted and prompted to contact the Regional Ambulance Center in a bid to establish why there is no immediate response. He is also able to assign specific ambulances to the mission. For example, if there is an event on Gulf Road near Kuwait Towers and ambulance #20 is noticed nearby, he is at liberty to assign the same to the event. The entire process is practically instant since the objective is to get help to the scene within 8 minutes.

Away from Call Takers and Dispatchers are supervisors who are also stationed in the emergency room. Their work is to monitor all the calls taking place. They see to it that everyone is performing their duties to the letter and ensure the Call Takers' diagnosis on events is accurate. The entire system is referred to as the Computer Aided Dispatch System. It was

developed by a local firm called CyberMark or Intergraph Kuwait. The system stands out as the

most advanced in the entire Gulf region (Walters, 2008). Not even that of Dubai can get close.

This knowledge leads to the inference that Kuwait's medical service emergency system is indeed

well prepared to handle mass casualties. It is the best in the region in terms of technological

advancement and efficiency. A very helpful feature of the ambulances is that they are able to get

real time updates as may be informed by the caller. This is because the Call Taker sees to it that

all information of interest that is received from the ground is updated live on the screens in the

ambulances (M'Hallah, & Alkhabbaz, 2013). Another advanced feature is that once patients

have been picked up by the ambulances, paramedics fill up a digital form, listing every step of

the diagnosis.

The medical emergency system in Kuwait remains largely successful due to other efforts

away from the emergency rooms. In this breath, one finds need to mention the regular seminars

and workshops on medical emergency. They have remained integral in improving general

preparedness for disaster. They are indeed high profile and therefore regarded highly. Examples

are those given by American doctors where paramedics are enlightened on a number of subjects.

Notably, paramedics in the Kuwait system are not only Kuwaitis, rather are of different

nationalities.

The situation was worse in Kuwait before but much has improved. It has become

increasingly appreciated that the terrorism threat is real. Terrorists could be targeting Western

expatriates or their interests but when they strike, everyone is affected. The implication here is

that no one is immune. The country's national health care plan focuses on major expansion of the

healthcare system (World Health Databook, 2011). Today, the healthcare system is on one of the most modern in the world. Development of the health care infrastructure is a duty performed by the public sector, although the private sector is also getting involved.

Kuwait's health care system is mainly built upon primary care principles with primary, secondary, as well as tertiary delivery. A robust system has been developed with a clear vision to providing care that covers diseases as well as events that could result in mass casualties. Presently, the country has 92 health care centers spread throughout its territory and ensuring everyone in the country's six regions gets help when they need it (Walters, 2008). If an explosive goes off in any part of the country, or a building collapses, the mechanisms discussed above as employed by the EMS become useful in preventing fatalities or deaths. A major boost to the system is the presence of an expatriate workforce who offers training as well as direct services. It may also be imperative to note that the United Nations is significantly present in the country. A number of Affiliate Organizations of the UN have offices in Kuwait and they offer technical and financial assistance where needed. The World Health Organization has set specific priorities and works in collaboration with the Kuwaiti government to among other things improve governance, reform the health care system, review and/or strengthen legislation on health, and address decentralization of health services. There is also a major objective to improve delivery in the system by generally strengthening health care, programs of accreditation, as well as support national capacity building.

Concerned authorities within Kuwait are also working towards the upgrading of the country's referral system. Areas of information and operational research have also not been ignored. As such, the country has developed a comprehensive, consolidated, and integrated health information system as evidenced by the EMS scenario highlighted in this construction. A lot has been done in ensuring preparedness and effective response plan to deal with probable natural disasters besides emergencies like terror attacks. In the same regard, the EMS is the country's first aid squad, rescues squad, emergency squad, life squad, ambulance service, and ambulance squad. Emergency services revolve around it. EMS personnel are specially trained to offer the said services and every effort made to ensure that the facilities needed are availed at their disposal (Walters, 2008). It is appreciated that during emergencies, lives of people depend on how quick the EMS response is. The medical technicians and paramedics who are always standing by are integral in ensuring that mass casualties are minimized even in the event of terror attacks.

As Kuwait continues to play its role against terror, the risk of attack goes up by the day. However, the manner of health organization discussed is a source of relief since the system is quite sufficiently prepared to respond accordingly. One can be assured of swift response irrespective of the place or nature of an event. In as much as what has been done is adequately appreciated, one thinks the situation could be better with more government funding to the health care system. More private sector involvement would also ensure that efforts to reduce mass casualties yield more fruit.

References

Abbas, A. R. (January 01, 1999). *EMS in Kuwait*. Emergency Medical Services.

Alexander, Y. (2007). *Middle East terrorism: Current threats and future prospects*. Aldershot:
Dartmouth.

Boghard, L. P. (2006). *Kuwait amid war, peace and revolution: 1979-1991 and new challenges*.
Basingstoke, [England: Palgrave Macmillan.

Cordesman, A. H., & Gold, B. (2014). *The Gulf Military Balance: The Conventional and
Asymmetric dimensions*. Lanham: Center for Strategic & International Studies.

M'Hallah, R., & Alkhabbaz, A. (March 01, 2013). Scheduling of nurses: A case study of a
Kuwaiti health care unit. *Operations Research for Health Care*, 2, 1-19.

Terril, W. A., & Army War College (U. S). (2007).*Kuwaiti national security and the US-Kuwaiti
strategic relationship after Saddam*. Carlisle Barracks, PA: Strategic Studies Institute,
U.S. Army War College.

Walters, E.M. (January 01, 2008). *Health care in Kuwait*. Nursing Times, 75, 1.)

World Health Databook. (2011). London: Euromonitor Intl.

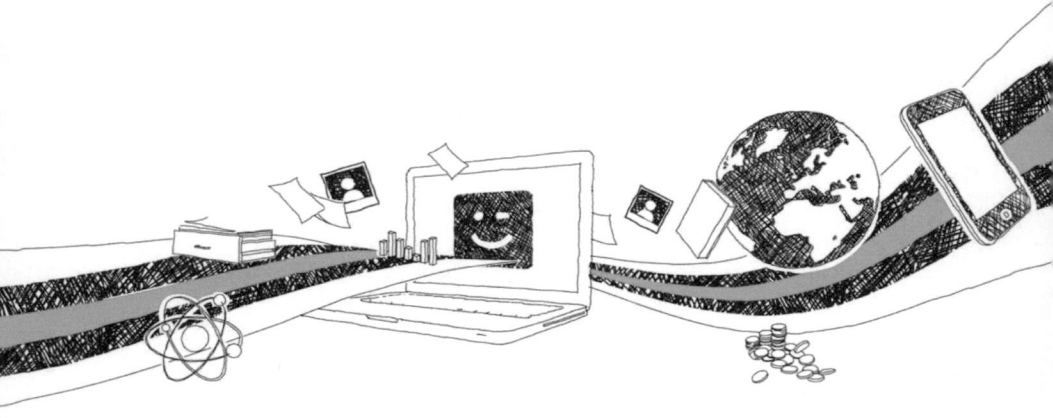
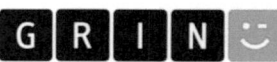